CBD

THE ULTIMATE OIL FOR PAIN

THE COMPLETE GUIDE TO THE RELIEF OF PAIN, ANXIETY, INSOMNIA, AND MUCH MORE FOR BETTER HEALTH WITHOUT THE HARMFUL SIDE EFFECTS

Disclaimer

The information contained in "CBD: The Ultimate Oil for Pain" and its components, is meant to serve as a comprehensive collection of strategies that the author of this eBook has done research about. Summaries, strategies, tips and tricks are only recommendations by the author, and reading this eBook will not guarantee that one's results will exactly mirror the author's results.

The author of this Ebook has made all reasonable efforts to provide current and accurate information for the readers of this eBook. The author and its associates will not be held liable for any unintentional errors that may be found.

The material in the Ebook may include information by third parties. Third party materials comprise of opinions expressed by their owners. As such, the author of this eBook will not assume responsibility or liability for any third party material or opinions.

The publication of third party material does not constitute the author's guarantee of any information, products, services, or opinions contained within third party material. Use of third party material does not guarantee that your results will mirror our results. Publication of such third party material is simply a recommendation and expression of the author's own opinion of that material.

Whether because of the progression of the Internet, or the unforeseen changes in company policy and editorial submission guidelines, what is stated as fact at the time of this writing may become outdated or inapplicable later.

This Ebook is copyright © 2019 with all rights reserved. It is illegal to redistribute, copy, or create derivative works from this Ebook whole or in parts. No parts of this report may be reproduced or retransmitted in any form whatsoever without the written, expressed and signed permission from the author.

Medical Disclaimer

All content published in this book is for informational purposes only. It is not intended to be a substitute for professional medical advice and should not be relied on as health or personal advice.

Always seek the advice of your doctor or other qualified health professional with any questions you may have regarding your health or a medical condition. Never disregard the advice of a medical professional, or delay in seeking it because of something you have read in this book.

You assume full responsibility for how you choose to use the information contained in this book.

TABLE OF CONTENTS

Note from the author:

In 2016 I was diagnosed with Crohn's disease. However, that was after 14 years of symptoms, multiple doctor visits and many misdiagnoses. I had several tests ran including an MRI, CT Scan, upper GI and 3 lower GI's. It wasn't until I was hospitalized in October 2016 that I first heard of Crohn's disease.

My husband and I started researching the disease before I even left the hospital. I was relieved when I found out that it isn't fatal, although it is considered an autoimmune disease that is accompanied by severe pain. With that said, there were many times that I thought the pain was worse than death. With all the pain that Crohn's induces, it is also a humiliating disease due to the fact that you are making several trips to the bathroom a day not knowing if you're going to make it to the toilet in time. It's really difficult to explain this disease unless you have this disease or know someone that does. I followed the doctor's advice and started taking Humira, which suppresses your immune system. The injections are expensive and painful. After about 6 months they quit working, if they ever worked at all. I was told to continue taking them even though the side effects where seriously dangerous. I continued to take them for another four months until I landed back in the emergency room. That was it! I was done! My husband and I decided to start researching natural methods of treatment, like Mangosteen and Curcumin. They helped for a time but didn't alleviate all the symptoms. Finally, we found CBD!

This book is the result of many long hours researching CBD and the benefits that come with taking it. At first, I was very skeptical of the many testimonials I seen. But after so many, you have to start to ask yourself, why wouldn't it work for me? I began to have a glimmer of hope that there was something out there, something more than just what the doctors prescribe. Don't get me wrong, CBD is not a cure all! But I do believe that, when taken properly and consistently, CBD can and does place my Crohn's in remission.

INTRODUCTION

You hear about it in the media, and you'll see it in your neighborhood store; Cannibidiol, also known as CBD, is rapidly becoming one of the best supplements worldwide and for good reason. With this recent increase in popularity, it is no wonder that many of us want to know more about what makes this special compound so amazing.

What is CBD? Why has it become so famous, and why only recently? Is it safe? Is it pleasant to ingest? Is it for me? I'm sure you have a hundred such questions. This is exactly why this book was written: To help people like you understand CBD and grasp its potential power and benefits.

CBD is often overshadowed by THC, which provides many of the effects most commonly associated with cannabis. THC is the compound responsible for the psychoactive effects of marijuana, causing what is known as a "high."

CBD, on the other hand, is actually non-psychoactive. It's legal, and, in fact, even has some opposite effects to those of THC. Cannabidiol can improve overall wellness, increasing your quality of life in a similar way to medicinal marijuana but without the high, offering relaxation and calm.

The THC in marijuana, as you might well know, used to be an illegal substance in most states. Marijuana has become synonymous with crime and addiction in the minds of many until recently. Studies have started to reveal that marijuana may actually become a source of hope and relief for people who need it most. Marijuana has been shown to help both healthy and ill individuals feel more relaxed and enjoy an overall better quality of life.

CBD was found to be one of the main cannabinoids showing promise as a relaxing and wellness-inducing substance. Even better, CBD did not cause psychotropic effects, which made it absolutely legal.

Yet, despite all this evidence - and because of the common abuse of its psychoactive effects - marijuana remains illegal for the general public in a select few states.

This is where industrial hemp and CBD can help. You wonder what industrial hemp actually is? Well, you are not alone!

Industrial hemp has been cultivated since ancient times in Eastern Asian countries for its oil and its strong fibers, which were used to make cloth. In ancient China, hemp seed oil was considered medicinal on top of being a great source of nutrition. Much later, that same interest in CBD oil began to grow in the West.

When processed correctly, industrial hemp seed and stalk oil contains only tiny traces of THC but a significant amount of CBD. This makes it ideal for making high-grade CBD supplements.

Legal and certified shops, whether it be a brick and mortar store in your local city or a reputable online seller, offer you the highest-quality CBD products in a variety of forms that will simply amaze you.

WHAT IS CANNABIDIOL (CBD)?

CBD is the acronym for cannabidiol and is the second-most abundant cannabinoid in the hemp plant and has many potential therapeutic benefits, including anti-inflammatory, analgesic, anti-anxiety and seizure-suppressant properties just to name a few. It can be sourced from both marijuana plants and hemp plants, which are legal in most countries as they contain minor amounts of THC.

CBD is one of the most well-known chemical compounds found inside the cannabis plant aside from THC. Unlike THC however, CBD does not produce the psychoactive effect that has become commonly associated with marijuana nor many of the other symptoms. In other words, they are both cannabinoids, but one is distinctly separate from THC meaning that they are different substances. CBD is also extremely famous for its ability to reduce the side effects of THC.

Because of its non-psychoactive effects and great potential healing properties, cannabidiol holds an exceptionally high medicinal value that will be paramount in how we treat medical conditions moving forward. It has uni□ue traits that make it stand out as an excellent treatment for a variety of conditions, symptoms, and diseases.

CBD is found in both hemp and cannabis

Hemp is a variety of the Cannabis Sativa plant that is grown for the industrial use of its fiber. Its history dates back over 10,000 years and is used to provide the raw material for textiles, biodegradable plastics, rope, nutraceuticals, construction materials, biofuel, food and more. Hemp is a tall, non-psychoactive plant, containing low levels of THC.

Note: For the purposes of this book, "marijuana" and "cannabis" will be used interchangeably even though we know that hemp is also a cannabis plant.

At the time the Controlled Substances Act of 1970 went into effect, it was illegal to grow industrial hemp in the United States. However, hemp products that were legally sold in the US had to meet three criteria:

- The hemp could not originate in the U.S.
- It must've been lawfully imported
- The material must've been derived from the "mature stalks and seeds" or "oil and cake made from seeds" of industrial hemp plants.

CBD products sold in states where medical/recreational marijuana is legal can extract CBD from either industrial hemp or a CBD-rich strain of cannabis. However, there are notable differences between CBD derived from cannabis versus hemp.

The synergy of the different compounds in cannabis work together to produce therapeutic effects on the body that are not achieved by the compounds individually. Essentially, the compounds work better together in what is known as the 'entourage effect.' Because of this, CBD derived from cannabis can be more effective when administered with higher levels of THC and terpenes. The mixture of the compounds accentuates the desired effects of cannabinoids on the body. For example, clinical research has shown that a 1:1 ratio of CBD to THC is effective for neuropathic pain.

As a whole, industrial hemp still contains less CBD than CBD-rich cannabis strains and lacks the robust terpene and cannabinoid profile that cannabis provides. Large amounts of industrial hemp are required to extract a small amount of CBD oil, raising questions about contaminants. Hemp is a bioaccumulator, meaning it draws toxins from the soil that could potentially end up in the extracted oil. This is one reason you want to make sure that the brand of CBD you decide to purchase has been properly tested.

CBD is best extracted from the flower and leaves, and only to a minor extent, the stalk of the hemp plant.

CBD oil and products that are obtained from the Cannabis sativa plant or more specifically, industrial hemp, contain high amounts of CBD and only trace amounts THC.

This means that hemp extract containing hemp CBD is ideal for those wishing to harness its powerful effects. Other hemp products include hemp oil, which is a healthy addition to a balanced diet and a nurturing addition to skincare and hair products.

How CBD works?

Despite the fact that there are all kinds of studies and intense research is being performed about the ways that CBD works in the body, this is not entirely clear yet. What scientists do know for a fact is that CBD, just like THC, causes a broad range of effects in our bodies by interacting with the endocannabinoid system which includes two types of cannabinoid receptors: CB1 and CB2.

CB1 receptors can be found in many areas of the brain, and they play an essential role in functions such as mood, memory, sleep, pain sensation, and appetite.

CB2 receptors are usually found in the immune system are they are responsible for cannabis' anti-inflammatory effects.

Endocannabinoids (cannabinoids produced by the body) typically activate both CB1 and CB2 receptors, and the main endocannabinoids that are found in our body are anandamide and arachidonoyl glycerol. The Endocannabinoid System is a vital system in the human body, which has receptors spread out across the entire organism, with higher concentrations in the brain and immune system. This system has evolved to specifically manage the effects of cannabinoids in the body, such as THC and CBD.

When CBD enters the body, the ECS receptors pick up on these compounds and immediately react and start regulating and managing them to where they are most needed and can do the most good. By sending these compounds in the areas of the body which need them the most, the ECS is actively working to induce a state of balance in the organism, and boost overall health.

With receptors all over the human body, the Endocannabinoid System controls vital functions such as pain, inflammation, sleep, mood, memory, appetite, and more. When you stimulate the Endocannabinoid System with CBD supplements, it will, in turn, regulate and improve vital functions in your body, with little to no health risks or side effects.

THC mimics the effects of the body's endocannabinoids by also activating both CB1 and CB2 receptors. But, unlike THC, CBD doesn't seem to act directly on cannabinoid receptors. Instead, it works indirectly on them, and it boosts the levels of endocannabinoids in the body. CBD can stimulate the release of endocannabinoids, and it also interferes with their natural breakdown.

Main effects of CBD

- Anti-depressant: It combats anxiety and depression.
- Anti-convulsant: It suppresses seizure activity.
- Anti-oxidant: It fights neuro-degenerative disorders.
- Anti-psychotic: It combats psychosis.
- Neuro-protective: It protects the neurons in the brain.
- Anti-emetic: It reduces nausea and vomiting.
- Anti-inflammatory: It combats inflammation and also the pain.
- Anti-tumoral: It combats tumor and cancer cells.

How THC works?

When THC penetrates the brain, it stimulates the cells to release the substance called dopamine, and it also activates the cannabinoid receptors which affect the brain in various ways. The initial state will be a relaxed one combined with a mellow feeling. The eyes may dilate, and other senses will be enhanced. More reported effects include a mix of emotions such as happiness and elation, unease and anxiety, relaxation and pain relief.

When cannabis is smoked, the THC (tetrahydrocannabinol) enters the bloodstream and makes its way to the brain where it interferes with receptors. The largest numer of these receptors reside in the par of the brain that controls pleasure, memory, concentration, sensory experiences, time perception, learning and coordination.

THC will also change the way we think. It can also cause hallucinations and delusions. The immediate effects usually start within 10 to 30 minutes after THC consumption.

Main effects of THC

- Analgesic: It relieves pain and inflammation.
- Relaxation: It creates a state of relaxation and well-being.
- Drowsiness: It induces sleep.
- Euphoria: It causes the state of "high."
- Appetite stimulant: It creates the urge to eat.

The psychoactive/psychological effects of THC include the following: time distortion, intensified sensory experiences, increased socialization.

CBD lacks all these harmful cognitive effects featured by THC, and in fact, it can even counteract the psychoactive effects of THC when administered from the extract and in plant form.

Medicinal properties of CBD

As you can see, CBD has "multiple targets of action," meaning that it works at many different places, giving it numerous medicinal properties, which include:

- Potent anti-inflammatory
- Antioxidant
- Neuroprotectant
- Anticonvulsant
- Analgesic (pain reliever)
- Anxiolytic (anti-anxiety)
- Antidepressant
- Antipsychotic
- Antispasmodic
- Anti-cancer agent

CBD modulates the intoxicating effects of THC and reduces the adverse effects that some people experience with THC, namely rapid heartbeat, anxiety, and short-term memory loss. At the same time, when CBD is taken with THC to treat pain, the combination reduces pain more significantly than THC alone. In low doses, CBD is described as alerting. In high doses it can be sedating. Amazingly, CBD has very little side effects even at high doses.

Common health benefits of CBD

Scientific research shows the many health benefits of CBD. Even despite CBD being a component of marijuana, it does not produce the psychoactive effects that have made marijuana attractive for recreational use. CBD benefits are real because CBD produces strong medicinal and therapeutic effects for even the most common conditions.

Digestive Aid

A healthy appetite is vital to a healthy body, especially when the body is healing. Some illnesses decrease the appetite to the point of preventing the body from healing itself. CBD stimulates appetite, according to the National Cancer Institute. In the human body, CBDs bind to cannabinoid receptors in the body. Scientists believe these receptors play an important role in regulating feeding behavior.

CBD also eases nausea and vomiting. This is especially helpful for individuals enduring chemotherapy and other treatments for serious diseases.

Analgesic

CBDs affect the CB1 receptors in the body to relieve pain. CBD also has an anti-inflammatory effect that reduces swelling that would be associated with the CB2 receptor.

Anxiety Relief

CBD may alleviate severe social anxiety. Generalized Social Anxiety Disorder (SAD), is one of the most common forms of anxiety disorders that impair quality of life. Some consumers complain of increased social anxiety after marijuana use, but this may be due to low levels of CBD proportionate to the higher levels of THC.

Scientists wanted to study the effects of CBD on people with SAD. The scientists selected 24 people with this condition who had never received treatment for SAD, then divided participants into two groups. One group received 600 mg of CBD while the control group received a placebo. The scientists then asked study participants to take part in a simulated public speaking test while researchers measured blood pressure, heart rate and other measurements of physiological and psychological stress.

The CBD group showed significantly reduced anxiety, cognitive impairment and discomfort in their speech performance. In comparison, those in the placebo group presented higher anxiety, cognitive impairment and discomfort.

According to the National Institute of Mental Health, approximately 15 million adults in the United States have social phobia and about 6.8 million have a generalized anxiety disorder. Traditional treatment usually involves counseling and medications. Treatment with CBD may be better than anti-depressants because it acts quickly and does not cause side effects or withdrawal symptoms.

Cancer Spread

The National Cancer Institute details several studies into the anti-tumor effects of CBD. One study in mice and rats suggest CBDs "may have a protective effect against the development of certain types of tumors." CBDs may do this by inducing tumor cell death, inhibiting cancer cell growth, and by controlling and inhibiting the spread of cancer cells.

One study by California Pacific Medical Center suggests CBD "turns off" the gene involved in the spread of breast cancer. These scientists found CBD inhibits ID-1, an action that prevents cancer cells from traveling long distances to distant tissues.

How does CBD interact with the body?

All of the 60 plus cannabinoids unique to the plant genus cannabis, interact with our bodies through the endocannabinoid system.

If you recall, the endocannabinoid system runs throughout your body. It's loaded with receptors that bind to the cannabinoids you introduce to your bloodstream when you consume cannabis. It's the chemical interactions of those bonds that create a wide and largely unknown series of responses in your body.

And even though CBD has no psychoactivefor humans, meaning, it doesn't make you intoxicated (i.e. high), it is highly reactive with the endocannabinoid system.

To put things as simply as possible, CBD makes things happen. When it interacts with the endocannabinoid system's receptors, it stimulates all kinds of changes in the body.

Where does CBD come from?

Cannabis plants come in a variety of strains. Each strain produces a particular balance of cannabinoids. Cannabinoids can account for as much as 25% or more of the content of the flowers. The amount of cannabinoids a plant can produce is limited, so as one cannabinoid is bred into a strain, the others are bred out. So, there are strains that are high in THC and low in CBD, and others that are high in CBD and low in THC, and some plants have more of a balance of the two.

Some strains of hemp are bred to be high in CBD and extremely low in THC. The essential oil extracts of cannabis flowers contain cannabinoids in the same ratio as the plant from which it is extracted, therefore, hemp extracts contain negligible amounts of THC.

Hemp is also far cheaper to grow and process than marijuana, so quite often, the CBD in CBD-infused products is extracted from hemp rather than marijuana and refined into CBD-rich essential oils and pure CBD. In order for a patient to be sure that their medicine is 100% THC-free, only hemp-derived products should be used. Note: Hemp plants do contain trace amounts of THC (<0.3%).

How is CBD made?

In order to extract CBD from the hemp plant, the flowers and leaves are ground up and soaked in a solvent of some kind (ethanol, supercritical CO_2, etc.) which separates the essential oils from the plant matter. The resulting product is correctly referred to as hemp extract. This extract will contain cannabinoids and other oily compounds found in the plant such as terpenes in the same ratio as the plant.

The next step in producing CBD is to concentrate the extract using a distillation process. This removes some of the unwanted contents and produces CBD concentrate. The resulting ratio of CBD and other compounds depends on the process and how many steps of distillation it has gone through.

CBD concentrate can also be further refined to produce CBD isolate, which can be as high as 99% pure CBD. CBD isolate takes on a salt-like crystal form at room temperature.

CBD concentrates and CBD isolates can be consumed by themselves, or they can be added to vegetable oils such as hemp seed oil, coconut oil, olive oil, and so on, as well as non-plant-based oils such as emu oil. These preparations can be used both internally and topically.

IS CBD LEGAL?

Is CBD legal? This is the most common, and most misunderstood, question surrounding this subject. There used to be a time that CBD and THC were both classified by the Drug Enforcement Agency (DEA) as Schedule 1 drug at the federal level. That means that the US federal government classified these two substances under the same schedule that includes Heroin, LSD, and Ecstacy, just to name a few of the more common ones.

The history of cannabis goes back thousands of years and is an excellent subject for future writings, but we're going to concentrate on the part of history when cannabis first started being regulated in the United States.

Here's a timeline to help you better understand some of the contemporary history of cannabis:

- Up until 1906 – Cannabis, including hemp, was a primary crop grown by thousands of farmers including some of our forefathers like George Washington, Thomas Jefferson, and John Adams.
- 1906 – Restrictions started increasing.
- 1920s – Prohibitions began.
- Mid – 1930s - Cannabis was being regulated as a drug in every state, not to mention the 35 states that adopted the Uniform State Narcotic Drug Act which

was primarily to produce revenue for the federal government.

- 1937 – First regulation of cannabis came about with the Marihuana Tax Act of 1937.
- 1970 – The Controlled Substances Act of 1970 was officially passed and formally outlawed the use of cannabis for any use, including medical.

On December 20, 2018, President Donald Trump signed into law the Agriculture Improvement Act of 2018 (more commonly known as the 2018 Farm Bill). The 2018 Farm Bill, which went into effect on January 1, 2019, contains a broad range of provisions but among them are the legalization of the cultivation and sale of hemp. As a result of the 2018 Farm Bill, hemp is no longer classified as a Schedule 1 substance. Keep in mind that the Farm Bill is a federal statute and only legalizes hemp (and as a result, CBD made from hemp) at the federal level. So, while CBD is legal under Federal Law, it is always prudent to check your local laws.

The best way for manufacturers to avoid legal issues is to extract the CBD from hemp rather than cannabis. Some stores use industrial hemp grown by US farmers and processed in pharmaceutical grade facilities.

In the United States, any variety of cannabis with a THC concentration of not more than 0.3% is considered to be 'industrial hemp.' So as long as the CBD that you're using comes from hemp and contains less than 0.3% THC, you shouldn't have any concerns.

States where CBD is legal for recreational use

As of the writing of this book there are 10 states where the cannabis plant, including both marijuana and hemp are completely legal for recreational and medicinal use. These states, including Washington DC, are:

- Alaska
- California
- Colorado
- Maine
- Massachusetts
- Michigan
- Nevada
- Oregon
- Vermont
- Washington

So if you find yourself in one of these awesome states, you are free to legally use CBD in any form without regard to THC levels and without a prescription.

States where CBD is legal for medicinal use

In addition to the ten states that have legalized recreational marijuana, there are 23 other states that it is legal, but only at the medicinal level. These states include:

- Arizona

- Arkansas
- Connecticut
- Deleware
- Florida
- Hawaii
- Illinois
- Louisiana
- Maryland
- Minnesota
- Missouri
- Montana
- New Hampshire
- New Jersey
- New Mexico
- New York
- North Dakota
- Ohio
- Oklahoma
- Pennsylvania
- Rhode Island
- Utah
- West Virginia

We just listed a total of 33 states that some form of marijuana is legal and as a result, CBD as well. There are a total of 14 states that have some form of legal CBD at the medicinal level that doesn't fall into a list as nicely as the states listed above. They are:

- **Alabama** – The only way to get CBD legally in Alabama is to be a part of a state sponsored clinical trial or have a debilitating medical condition.

- **Georgia** – A patient can have CBD prescribed in Georgia providing the patient has at least one of over a dozen medical conditions. These medical conditions include cancer, Parkinson's disease, multiple sclerosis, and seizure disorders. The patient can't have more than 20 ounces of oil. The oil cannot be more than 5% THC and the CBD content must be greater than or equal to the THC content. In otherwords, for CBD oil to be legal in Georgia, it must contain at least as much CBD as it does THC.

- **Indiana** – Early in 2018, Indiana moved away from only allowing citizens that was on its patient registry to buy and use CBD oil. On March 21, 2018, the Governor of Indiana signed into law Senate Enrolled Act 52, which legalized the manufacturing, retail sell, and use of CBD oil provided it did not exceed 0.3% THC content in it.

- **Iowa** – The Department of Public Health will allow patients to use limited amounts of CBD oil as long as they are suffering from a predetermined list of medical conditions such as cancer, HIV/AIDS, seizures, and ALS.

- **Kansas** – An adult in Kansas can legally purchase, possess, and use CBD products as long as it doesn't contain any THC whatsoever.

- **Kentucky** – Even though there is growing support for the legalization of marijuana and CBD at least at the medical level, Kentucky can't seem to break away from the legislation they passed in 2014 which revised the definition of marijuana to create legal protection for patients who use CBD.

- **Mississippi** – The current CBD laws in Mississippi was adopted in 2014. The law makes it legal for patients with severe epilepsy to use CBD. The extract must have more than 15% CBD and no more than 0.5% THC. Patients that are prescribed CBD in Mississippi must consume it under the supervision of a licensed physician.
- **North Carolina** – North Carolina does have a medical cannabis program set to end in 2021 if studies fail to show and prove the benefits of CBD. As it stands now, patients with intractable epilepsy have access to low THC hemp extract.
- **South Carolina** – CBD is legal only to those patients suffering from severe epilepsy. The extract must be at least 15% CBD and no more than 0.9% THC.
- **Tennessee** – Again, only patients diagnosed with intractable epilepsy may be prescribed a CBD extract. It must not contain more than 0.9% THC. Only CBD extracted fromfrom the hemp plant is legal in Tennessee.
- **Texas** – The Compassionate Use Act only allows patients diagnosed with epileptic seizures by a doctor who specializes in epilepsy to prescribe CBD. The CBD extract prescribed must not have more than 0.5% THC. The caveat is, the patient must try two current FDA approved epilepsy drugs before they can be prescribed CBD.
- **Virginia** – CBD oil is legal for any patient who has any condition that has been diagnosed by a licensed doctor or practitioner.
- **Wisconsin** – In 2014 CBD was only legal to treat seizure disorders. In 2017, the Wisconsin Senate

expanded the legal parameters to include the treatment of any medical condition a doctor has recommended it for.

Wyoming – CBD is only legal for patients with epilepsy. Again, the patient must not have responded favorably to other treatments. Even then, a neurologist must plead a case with the Wyoming Department of Health on how CBD would in fact help the patient. The extract will be high concentrations of CBD with trace amounts of THC.

The push to legalize cannabis started in 1996 when California voted to legalize it for medicinal purposes. To date, a total of 47 states have adopted legal cannabis laws of some sort, ranging from purchasing CBD with zero THC to full legalization of recreational marijuana and everything in between. Three states still haven't adopted any laws allowing adults to purchase cannabis in any way, shape, or form. They are:

- Idaho
- South Dakota
- Nebraska

State and federal laws are constantly changing around cannabis. If you live in a state where the cannabis laws are a little gray, I highly recommend you familiarize yourself with the laws of your state.

DOES CBD GET YOU HIGH?

There are dozens of chemicals in the cannabis flower that have very different effects; some of them have no real effect, but others can change your perception on the way medical marijuana is used.

CBD and THC are the most popular known cannabinoids which form a group of chemical compounds that are naturally produced only by cannabis plants. Both CBD and THC exist in the crystalline resinous trichomes that cover the mature cannabis flower, and both of them are the cannabinoids that we find most abundantly in marijuana. But each strain produces different amounts of the compounds. They share the same chemical formula with the only difference is that their atoms are arranged in a variety of ways, but they have widely different effects on our body because they interact with our endocannabinoid system differently.

CBD does not get you high. In fact, when taken with THC, CBD actually reduces just how high you can get. Here's the science behind why CBD won't get you high and how it takes the edge off the high produced by THC.

Think of THC and CBD as batteries. THC is a AA, and CBD is a AAA. The CB1 receptor in your brain only turns on when the right size battery is inserted, in this case, the AA

(THC). The AA fits nicely into the receptor, turns it on, and produces the psychoactive high that we have all heard of and/or experienced.

But the AAA (CBD) also fits into the receptor. It's not an exact match like the AA, so the AAA doesn't activate the receptor. That's why CBD doesn't get you high: it's not built to activate the receptors that cause your world to go psychedelic.

So now you've got an AAA battery occupying a space made for an AA battery. If an AA battery comes along, it's going to "bounce off" that receptor because the AAA battery is already there. That's how CBD can take the edge off the high caused by THC: the CBD molecule reduces the chances that THC will activate the CB1 receptors. In essence, it's a clash between cannabinoids.

ARE THERE ANY RISKS OR SIDE EFFECTS?

Although, side effects are very rare to those consuming CBD, it's important to note that the impact of the few that do exist could be unwelcome. Take drowsiness for example. If taken in tandem with a medication that also causes drowsiness, patients who must be alert for work could be put at risk.

So far, CBD has not been shown to have any severe or fatal impact on patients in clinical trials. Here are a few of the minor CBD side effects that could be unwelcome for potential consumers of the medication.

Impacts on drug metabolism

The body produces a series of enzymes that help patients to consume and benefit from CBD. Use of CBD combined with other drugs can keep medications from being properly processed by the body.

In test trials, CBD has been shown to neutralize P450 enzyme activity in some patients. This is one of the main enzymes in the liver that helps to metabolize medications. This should remind patients to consult a physician or a pharmacist before adding any medications to their routine. It should be noted that grapefruits can also have this impact on the liver's metabolizing capabilities. So no need to panic if you've taken CBD in tandem with any medication. But it's important to check and see if your medication is still working. Complications like these can easily be worked out by rescheduling your medication at different times of the day. You can live with a reduced P450 enzyme for a short time as your body can reset the balance a few hours later.

Dry mouth

If you have issues with dehydration, CBD could exacerbate your problems. Some patients have reported CBD side effects that include an 'unpleasant dry sensation throughout the day.' As noted above, CBD has an effect on secretions of glands and this will include saliva. Cannabinoid receptors are present in the glands that produce saliva, which can lead to dry mouth. It's not too severe of an impact but can cause some amount of discomfort. Staying hydrated or drinking sports drinks with electrolytes can counteract this balance.

It could have the positive impact of getting some patients to drink more water than they normally would on a given day.

Increased tremors

For people who suffer from Parkinson's disease, CBD should not be taken in high doses. High doses in some early research has been shown to increase tremors for Parkinson's patients. Inflammation and pain related to Parkinson's can be treated with CBD. Many patients report positive impacts on the other effects of Parkinson's.

When taken in lower doses, CBD has been tested to having positive impacts on alleviating Parkinson's related pain. If you're taking CBD related to Parkinson's, your CBD side effects could be a dosage issue. Try lowering the dosage before discarding the treatment altogether. Always consult your doctor before beginning any treatment or changing your dosage.

Low blood pressure

As CBD slows down some of the body's processes during moments of inflammation or illness, it can also work to slow the process too much. CBD could cause a drop in blood pressure for some patients. It usually happens right after you administer the medication.

Low blood pressure can be an issue if you're recovering from surgery or any kind of accident. It also affects how uickly other medications will move through your system.

If you experience any of the lightheadedness often associated with low blood pressure, talk to a physician. It could be an effect of your CBD treatment or a drug interaction you may not have predicted.

As we've said before, the side effects associated with CBD are virtually non esistent to the vast majority of consumers using it. However, it's always a good idea to consult a medical professional before embarking on your first CBD journey.

WHAT ARE TERPENES?

Terpenes are basically the unsaturated hydrocarbons found in the essential oils of plants. They are found in different plants and even some insects. When you walk through a forest and smell the pine scent in the air, you are essentially smelling the terpene Pinene, which is responsible for giving you that uplifting feeling. Another example is the smell of lemon when you're polishing your furniture. The terpene Limonene can be thanked for that smell and the good mood that comes with it. Although there are literally hundreds of terpenes in nature, there are only about ten that really affect the world of cannabis. They are:

- Pinene
- Limonene
- Myrcene
- Linalool
- Delta-3-Carene
- Eucalyptol
- Caryophyllene
- Humulene
- Ocimene
- Terpineol

The following is an in depth look at the ten most commonly found terpenes in the cannabis plant. You will find that all these terpenes have an aroma associated with it, as well as certain health benefits, different vaporizing temperatures, various medicinal values, and different places to find each of them in nature.

A closer look at common terpenes in cannabis

Pinene

- Smells like pine
- Vaporizes at 311 degrees F.
- Used to treat asthma, pain, ulcers, anxiety, and cancer.
- Help with alertness, memory retention, and counteracts some THC effects.
- Can be found in pine needles, basil, parsley, dill, and rosemary.

Limonene

- Has a citrus smell to it.
- Vaporizes at 348 degrees F.
- Used to treat anxiety, depression, inflammation, pain, and cancer.
- Helps with reducing stress and has a tendency to elevate moods.
- Can be found in fruit rinds, rosemary, juniper, and peppermint.

Myrcene

- The terpene most prevalent in the cannabis plant.

- Concentration dictates whether a strain will have a sedative effect or an energetic effect.
- Cardamom, herbal, cloves, musky, and earthy are the aromas for Myrcene. Although a pleasant smell, not one that is used directly too often.
- Vaporizes at 332 degrees F.
- Used to treat insomnia, pain, inflammation, as well as a great antioxidant.
- Helps with relaxation and at levels of >0.5%, can have a sedating "couchlock" effect.
- Can be found in mango, lemongrass, thyme, and hops.

Linalool

- Has a floral smell
- Vaporizes at 388 degrees F.
- Used to treat anxiety, depression, insomnia, pain, inflammation, and neurodegeneration.
- Helps with sedation and mood enhancement.
- Found in lavender.

Delta-3-Carene

- Has a sweet, pungent, woody, pine, and cedar combination smell.
- Vaporizes at 338 degrees F.
- Used to treat depression, and is a good anti-inflammatory and antihistamine. Also used to dry out excess body fluids like sweat, tears, mucus, as well as menstrual flow.
- Helps with insomnia and improves memory.
- Can be found in pine, cedar, and rosemary.

Eucalyptol

- Has a camphor smell to it.
- Vaporizes at 349 degrees F.
- Used for Alzheimer's, asthma, bacteria, cancer, anti-oxidant, and anti-inflammatory.
- Helps with mental clarity and headaches.
- Can be found in eucalyptus, camphor laurel, bay leaves, tea tree, mugwort, sweet basil, wormwood, rosemary, and common sage.

Caryophyllene

- Smells like cloves and pepper as well as spicy and woody.
- Vaporizes at 266 degrees F.
- Used for pain, anxiety, depression, and ulcers.
- Helps with stress relief.
- Found in black pepper, cloves, and cinnamon.

Humulene

- Has a woody, earthy aroma with the smell of hops
- Vaporizes at 222 degrees F.
- Used primarily as an anti-inflammatory.
- Found in coriander, basil, cloves, and hops.

Ocimene

- Smells sweet, herbal, and woody.
- Vaporizes at 122 degrees F.
- Used for antiviral, antifungal, antibacterial, antiseptic, and a decongestant.
- Found in basil, mangoes, orchids, pepper, parsley, mint, and kumquats.

Terpineol

- Aroma is piney, floral, and herbal.
- Vaporizes at 366 degrees F.
- Used for cancer, fungus, bacteria, sedative, and an antioxidant.
- Has a sedating effect.
- Found in nutmeg, apples, conifers, tea tree, lilacs, and cumin.

Keep in mind that since CBD isolates are stripped down to just the CBD, they lack most, if not all, of the terpenes that is naturally found in the plant. I'm not saying that the CBD isolates are not a good option, especially if THC is a factor. What I am saying is that you can't get the entourage effect of the CBD through an isolate.

FULL SPECTRUM VS ISOLATE

Due to its non-psychoactive healing properties, CBD has become a very popular option for patients seeking a natural alternative to treat conditions such as chronic pain, anxiety, epilepsy, and more. As patients start to understand how CBD can be used to alleviate their symptoms, they are often faced with a choice between using products made from CBD isolate or full spectrum CBD.

Difference between CBD isolate vs full spectrum CBD

When CBD is referred to as full spectrum or whole plant CBD, it means that the CBD contains all the other cannabinoids found in the cannabis or hemp plant (about 85 total) including CBN (Cannabinol), CBG (Cannabigerol), and THCV (Tetrahydrocannabivarin), to name a few. THC and CBD are the ones we are most familiar with. Full spectrum CBD from hemp contains trace amounts of THC but in very low concentrations (up to 0.3%). Full spectrum CBD from the cannabis plant can contain significantly higher amounts of THC.

CBD isolate, on the other hand, is simply purified CBD that has been extracted from the cannabis or hemp plant and isolated from the other cannabinoids. So essentially, it's CBD in its purest form without any other cannabinoids to accompany it.

CBD isolate vs full spectrum CBD: Which is more effective?

It was previously believed that CBD in its isolated form was more potent and concentrated than full spectrum CBD. However, in 2015, the theory was debunked by a study from the Lautenberg Center for General Tumor Immunology in Jerusalem. In the study, researchers administered full spectrum CBD and CBD isolate to two different groups of mice. When comparing the data of the two groups, the results proved that the group administered with full spectrum CBD were provided with higher levels of relief. Furthermore, the study demonstrated that full spectrum CBD continued to provide relief as the dose increased, while CBD isolate did not provide the same effect when there was an increase in dosage.

While full spectrum CBD has ultimately proven to be more effective than CBD isolate and can be used to effectively treat a wide variety of ailments, it does not discredit the effectiveness of CBD isolate. There are a wide variety of situations when CBD isolate would be preferred over full spectrum CBD. For example, you may not necessarily need the full capabilities of full spectrum CBD, or if you aren't legally allowed to use THC. It is also important to note that other cannabinoids may cause negative reactions when isolated CBD wouldn't (if the condition you are suffering from is critical, we advise you speak to a medical consultant before trying out any version of CBD).

Products that advertise "whole plant CBD" are also good because they'll incorporate the entourage effect. The entourage effect refers to how cannabinoids and terpenes react with one another in the body. Research suggests that these compounds work best when combined together like they are naturally found in the marijuana plant, rather than if they are isolated in a lab. Therefore, whole plant CBD products are usually more effective than CBD isolates.

CBD AS AN ANTI-INFLAMMATORY

The anti-inflammatory properties of CBD come well documented. Reducing inflammation is a recognized potential use case for the diverse cannabinoid. Naturally, reducing inflammation helps to combat chronic inflammation. Believed to be the precursor to heart disease, diabetes, and several forms of cancer, chronic inflammation prevention is linked to living a longer, happier life.

In one study, they monitored the reaction between CBD and glycine receptors. The receptors were linked to dorsal horn neurons in the spines of rats. These are a collection of sensory neurons that transmit information, in this case telling our brain we are in pain. Researchers concluded that administration of CBD, significantly suppress chronic inflammatory and neuropathic pain.

A further study examined the effectiveness of CBD at mitigating inflammation. The study focussed on biopsies from patients with ulcerative colitis (UC) and intestinal segments of mice with LPS-induced intestinal inflammation. UC is a long-term chronic condition that causes the human colon and rectum to become inflamed. Again, CBD demonstrated its efficiency. Preliminary results showed that CBD counteracts the inflammatory environment induced by LPS in mice and also in human colonic cultures derived from UC patients.

CBD can reduce inflammation too much

Thankfully, that is something scientists at the Research Center of the University Institute of Cardiology and Pulmonology of Quebec also wanted to understand. An appropriate inflammatory response is vital for our immune system to be effective in fighting infections. By analysing data collated by the scientific community, the regulation of lung immunity and inflammation caused by cannabinoids was scrutinized.

Initial interpretation found that through the downregulation of the functions of immune cells, cannabinoids could diminish host defence. Doing so would increase the risk of contracting an infection, and reduce our immune system's effectiveness. They did go on to acknowledge that the relationship between too much and too little support with inflammation is a complicated one. More extensive research would be needed to transfer the data from animal models to humans.

Too much of a good thing can be bad

Conflicting research always makes for concerned reading. However, the inflammatory "balancing act" is no different from several other aspects of healthy living. If you take a look in your medicine cabinet, it is bound to be filled with a broad spectrum of health supplements. Iron, vitamin D, vitamin C; several essential supplements are needed to give our bodies a boost. It is a form of support that may be needed because of limitations in lifestyle or diet. Just like the scenario with CBD, ingesting too many vitamins can lead to adverse effects.

We shouldn't fear the implications of taking too much of something that is good for us. In most cases, the tolerable level is much higher when the effect is beneficial, rather than detrimental. In reality, something that is "good" for us can be "bad," and vice versa. The trouble is, if we segregate products in this way, it becomes impossible to know if a supplement is safe to consume. Instead, we should always come back to the theme of balance. Good versus bad is merely too basic, especially when each of us is uniquely different in our genetic makeup.

Dosage is crucial

We know from research that CBD has fantastic potential as a potent anti-inflammatory. We also know that in some of the data collected, this can lead to diminished effectiveness in our immune system. Presented with those two statements, the next logical step is to factor in dosage. The ideal dose of CBD will depend on numerous variables, more than have been studied thus far. Your physiology, the condition or disease, CBD concentration, external factors; the list of potential parameters is extensive.

While we wait for the experts to identify and narrow down variables, the safest option is to start low. Build CBD intake slowly to establish the impact on your own body. With a little patience, the hope is that comprehensive research will establish and quantify the exact implications of CBD use.

How can CBD be used as an anti-inflammatory drug?

Of all the qualities that CBD offers, it's anti-inflammatory properties are arguably the most well researched of the bunch. Being successfully utilized to treat almost all digestive conditions, as well as many other medical challenges, it is now looked upon as the most efficient anti-inflammatory drug available, even beating out traditional options such as Vitamin C and Omega 3 supplements!

It is important to have a good grasp on how CBD works with our bodies, though, in order to fully understand how it can be such a useful anti-inflammatory.

Like all cannabinoids, CBD interacts with our body upon consumption, but what is interesting about CBD is that it works differently to many of the other researched compounds of the plant, particularly when it comes to interaction with the endocannabinoid system.

If you recall, each and every one of us has an Endocannabinoid system (ECS), which has control over regulating many of our bodily functions and ensuring that everything runs smoothly. The ECS releases natural cannabinoids that are vital for a range of physiological things, from the way we think to the way we feel pain. In fact, it plays a part in almost every aspect of our being.

When CBD is consumed, it interacts with the ECS and encourages it to produce an increased number of natural cannabinoids. By doing this, our body is better able to heal and regulate various functions. Also, not only does CBD help produce self healing cannabinoids, but it also interacts with our CB2 receptors, which oversee our entire immune system.

CBD FOR PAIN RELIEF

If you're suffering from recurring aches or pains in your body, you know how frustrating it is. Maybe you're struggling through the constant cycle of waking up each morning stiff as a board, or worse yet, in the middle of the night. Is there any relief in sight? If it feels like you're in a constant state of popping anti-inflammatory pills like Aleve or Advil, you might find some relief with CBD oil.

Over the last few years, as CBD oil has become increasingly popular, it's being used to help with pain relief for people of all ages. The difference here is that CBD oil is non-psychoactive, so you're getting the medicinal benefits of cannabis without any of the physical "high."

A lot of medical studies back up the anecdotal claims for CBD's pain relief properties. CBD has properties that bind to the pain receptors within your body. This allows for the body to experience an alleviation in pain.

What causes pain?

Pain might seem to be a nuisance at times, but it is there to serve a purpose. Imagine touching a hot stove. It burns! This pain causes you to □uickly retract your finger from what is causing the pain, thereby protecting you. Cuts and scrapes and inflammation that come about from injuries also serve a purpose, with inflammation helping to protect a damaged area and remove pathogens from a wound, preventing infection. The central nervous system exists to alert us to such problems.

How is pain usually treated?

It was once advised that people suffering from chronic pain should stay in bed and rest, but we now know that this is probably the worst thing you can do. If your pain is muscular, such as might be the case with lower back pain, you must keep yourself moving, as staying still for long periods will only stiffen your muscles further. Staying in bed will also stop you from sleeping well, you will become lonely, the pain will get worse, and your other muscles and bones will weaken. It's just not worth it!

Instead, it is important to keep exercising through your pain. This isn't to say you should hit the gym and pump some iron. You can simply walk more, or take part in some swimming (where your weight will be taken by the water), peddle gently on an exercise bike, or engage in yoga. By all means, take and follow the advice of your doctor or physical therapist before working through your pain. But it is a common conception to exercise even despite chronic pain. Many believe that by strengthening the muscles of the body, you are better prepared to combat your pain.

However, this is generally not enough to rid people of chronic pain. Painkillers are extremely common for chronic pain, including over-the-counter medications like aspirin and ibuprofen. These types of medications aren't exactly good for you, though.

First of all, you will only be masking the pain and not solving any of the underlying problems. This is why painkillers such as these need to be taken every 4-6 hours to prevent the pain from returning. But it can be harmful to take these sorts of pharmaceuticals too much, as they can cause stomach ulcers and other damage to the body.

Stronger prescriptions are available for the most serious pains, and this even extends to opioids. Opiate painkillers are very strong and very effective at relieving pain, but they are also extremely addictive. There are literally thousands of overdoses each year in the US.

It's frightening that such a dangerous drug is so widely available for patients, and yet there are much safer and effective options such as CBD.

What type of pain can CBD help with?

We've seen people improve upon all types of pain issues, both chronic and acute pain types. Some of these pain sources include:

- Headaches – regular and migranes
- Muscle aches
- Back pain
- Joint pain
- Arthritis-related pain
- Inflammation relief

I'd like to make it abundantly clear: CBD oil is NOT a miracle cure. You have to give it a try to see if it'll work for you. Everyone's body chemistry is different. A reputable brand won't make outrageous claims about what it can do. It'll simply provide user testimonials and allow you to make the choice. Another important factor to take into consideration is the type of CBD you're using. Some people find that isolates provide the enough relief while others require a full spectrum CBD to find relief.

Although studies on CBD are being done daily, there is still a lot to learn about this very complex topic. With that said, the future is looking bright!

How does CBD work for pain relief?

Unfortunately, pain is a condition of human existence. Everybody experiences pain at one point or another whether it is from a trip or fall, a more serious accident, or if it is caused by an underlying condition, everybody feels pain.

Nowadays, people are looking for alternative methods to treat their aches and pains, as over the counter medications have a long list of drawbacks. Increasingly, CBD is being used for this very matter.

As we learned earlier, the human body contains a network of cannabinoid receptors and endocannabinoids (ones that we produce naturally). The endocannabinoid system works to keep our bodies functioning in a healthy manner by maintaining homeostasis, keeping our body in balance.

One of the functions that the ECS helps to regulate is pain and inflammation. It does this by 'listening' to conditions in the body through the cannabinoid receptors that sit on top of each cell. The receptors communicate this information to the inside of the cell, so that different parts of the body can respond accordingly. Hence, when injury occurs, the surrounding area is inflamed to protect it.

As we mentioned though, things can go wrong. If the inflammation persists, it is usually the job of endocannabinoids to stimulate their corresponding receptors to stop it, but this doesn't always happen.

By taking CBD, it is thought that you can indirectly influence the behavior of the ECS. CBD stimulates the production of more endocannabinoids, allowing you to give your body an added boost in times of need. In other words, taking CBD helps your body to work better, naturally.

A review carried out by Dr. Ethan Russo looked at studies ranging from the late 1980s all the way to 2007. Based on the results of these studies, it was concluded that CBD was effective in relieving overall pain without causing any adverse side effects. It was also noted that insomnia caused by chronic pain was relieved. Furthermore, those suffering from pain due to Multiple Sclerosis (MS) were most likely to benefit from CBD use.

From the studies that have been conducted so far, combined with anecdotal evidence from people already using CBD to relieve their pain, it seems that CBD could really offer some hope to people who have to deal with pain in their everyday lives.

CBD oil has a number of medical benefits

For example, studies show that CBD interacts with both your immune system and your brain receptors. These receptors receive a bunch of chemical signals from stimuli and help the rest of your cells respond to those signals. When your receptors react with CBD, they form anti-inflammatory effects that reduce pain.

CBD also helps treat conditions like anxiety, depression, fibromyalgia, and stress.

This makes CBD an effective treatment option for a multitude of medical conditions. But one of the biggest benefits of CBD is that it can help relieve symptoms of chronic pain.

CBD for Chronic Pain

As I've mentioned before, CBD has the ability to interact with the receptors that are found in your brain and also your immune system. So, for example, if you are suffering from chronic back pain, studies and numerous testimonials have have concluded that CBD can help tremendously. You can continuously take CBD oil for your chronic pain and not build up a tolerance to it. In other words, CBD oil provides a long term option for a long term problem. You don't have to keep increasing your dosage or search around for new medications that might work better.

Relieving of arthritis pain

Although many studies still need to be done to better understand painmanagement surrounding arthritis, a great number of arthritis patients have reported significant relief when takingCBD. As I've said before, CBD interacts with two receptors, which are the CB1 and CB2 receptors. The CB2 receptor plays an important role in the immune system and could help explain why CBD might be helpful in patients with inflammatory autoimmune forms of arthritis. A classic example is rheumatoid arthritis.

A recent study, conducted by researchers at the University of Kentucky, investigated the use of CBD in rats with arthritis. In the study, CBD was administered to rats for four consecutive days in the form of a gel, containing either 0.6, 3.1, 6.2, or 62.3 mg. The researchers noticed a reduction in inflammation and overall pain in the rats' arthritic joints, and no side effects were noted.

Cancer treatment

For those that has undergone chemotherapy, they always suffer from pain. But when you take in CBD, there is a good chance that you can manage the pain that might arise due to that painful process.

Relieving of acute pain

When we refer to acute pain, we are referring to pain that is brought on from cuts, infections and other kinds of physical injuries that you might get. Acute pain should come and go fast in a few hours, days, or weeks. But this is achievable if you are treated in the right way. As you've already learned, CBD has significant anti-inflammatory properties to it. Pain in general, including various types of acute pain, are caused by the inflammation of the tissue surrounding the injury. So, as a result, the anti-inflammatory properties of CBD can help acute pain.

Fibromyalgia pain

Fibromyalgia is a musculoskeletal disorder that causes pain and as a result, a lack of sleep, headaches, fatigue, depression, muscle pain, memory issues and mood concerns. Pain is a subjective feeling and sometimes it's hard to evaluate and measure it. But research has shown CBD to reduce pain and stiffness, enhance sleep, greater sensation of well-being, and also improvement of relaxation. CBD will give you more options for results with no side effects.

Diabetes pain

If you are suffering from type 1 or even type 2 diabetes, CBD has been shown to reduce inflammation as well as chronic inflammation. It also possesses properties that will improve resistance to insulin. Studies, as well as many testimonials of diabetics, have been shown to lower blood sugar levels, enhance the metabolism of the body and also manage pain from diabetes.

The benefits of using CBD oil for pain relief

- CBD has properties that has the ability to work with all types of pain.
- Capable of improving swelling, redness, reducing inflammation, and soreness.
- It can help you to avoid high doses of Ibuprofen, Oxytocin and also Percocet.

- You will not experience any liver or even kidney problems.
- If the CBD is in isolate form, the THC level will be so low that it probably will not even show on a drug test.
- There are virtually no side effects.
- It is not addictive.
- It is a natural product.

How to use CBD for pain relief?

There are several ways that you can use to take this product. Some of the ways include:

- You can ingest or swallow it.
- You can also take it under the tongue, a method known as sublingual.
- Consuming it with food or drinks.
- CBD is also available in creams which allow you to rub it on your skin.

A brighter future for pain

CBD is a legal compound that can be extracted from the cannabis plant, meaning that oil produced from it is legal to possess and use. More and more people are turning to CBD as a means of relieving symptoms of many conditions, with chronic pain being one of them.

A number of things can cause chronic pain, but no matter what the cause, it is possible that CBD could help. If you are tired of over the counter medications and the risks associated with them, CBD could be a natural way to sootheryour pain and tackle the underlying issue if that is inflammation.

CBD FOR ANXIETY.

Anxiety affects about 20% of Americans and comes in all shapes and sizes. There are clinical anxiety disorders like social anxiety, PSTD, and OCD, as well as everyday anxieties like trouble sleeping, tight deadlines, and fear of flying.

Many Americans with anxiety disorders are prescribed benzodiazepines like Xanax, Klonopin, and Valium, but these drugs are very addictive and make people feel lethargic and fuzzy.

Anti-anxiety medications have many side effects: cognitive deficits, unusual sleep behaviors, allergic reactions, impairment of driving, decreasing blood pressure, depression, loss of coordination, and increased risk of falling in the elderly. Unlike benzos, CBD has very few possible side effects, and of the few they do have, none are even close to the seriousness of the prescribed medications. Just think, a natural plant with very little possible side effects that produces a substance that helps sufferers with all the classic symptoms of anxiety, like racing thoughts, trouble sleeping, and difficulty being around people.

The other problem with benzodiazepines, they are dangerously addictive. In fact, benzo withdrawal is one of the only withdrawals that could potentially kill. The only other withdrawal as severe is alcohol. Even opioids are less "technically" addictive.

That's why so many people are choosing to quit the "hard stuff" and opt for something more natural, like CBD. In fact, according to a recent State of Cannabis Report by Eaze, 40% of cannabis consumers in California have completely replaced anxiety drugs with cannabis. What's more, of the 48% of respondents that said they use or have used anxiety medication, 95% of them said cannabis has helped them reduce their use of prescription anxiety pills. Those are very significant numbers.

However, because of benzos' highly addictive nature, replacing them with CBD should be done slowly and always, under a medical professional's supervision.

How CBD works for treating anxiety?

Again, CBD interacts with the body's own, natural endocannabinoid system (ECS). You'll notice that we often reference the ECS. The ECS is the core of everything that CBD is to the human body. The ECS is present in nearly "every cell in the body" and helps to regulate many of our bodies' functions, including:

- mood
- appetite
- sleep
- memory
- pain perception.

In fact, stress recovery is one of the endocannabinoid system's main purposes.

But what's more, researchers described how CBD also interacts with a neurotransmitter called GABA (gamma-aminobutyric acid). GABA transmits messages from one brain cell, or neuron, to another; that message is typically "slow down" or "stop firing." GABA tells the body when it's time to power down, and since millions of neurons in the brain respond to GABA, the effects include:

- reducing anxiety
- calming the nervous system
- helping with sleep
- relaxing the muscles.

"CBD is a GABA uptake inhibitor," says one researcher. "Meaning, it creates a surplus of GABA in the brain. That results in a quieting and calming effect. With CBD supplementation, patients don't have the racing thoughts that paralyze them at work or even lying awake in bed at night."

How to use CBD for anxiety?

Over the past few years, the variety of CBD products has grown exponentially. There are high CBD strains for smoking or vaping, like ACDC, Harlequin, and Charlotte's Web. A CBD vape pen is also an option, and there are a few specifically designed to relieve anxiety, like Dosist Calm, Select Oil's CBD collection, and Aya's Relax. Edibles high in cannabidiol are another popular choice for those wishing to use CBD for anxiety, like "Not Pot" CBD-only chocolates.

But one of the most popular ways to consume cannabidiol is still through CBD oil. Some of the best CBD oils include brands like Green Roads World and Pure CBD Vapors. They are especially good for anxiety because they contain little to no THC so there's no risk of getting "high." Cannabis oil can be added to food or simply dropped straight under the tongue for sublingual absorption, which kicks in the relief fast. Not to mention, CBD oil has no lingering smell, so medicating is totally discreet.

There are literally hundreds of brands and strains of CBD on the market today. Always do your own research before deciding which brand, strain, or type (full spectrum or isolate) of CBD to go with.

High CBD strains that will help calm your anxiety

Since CBD strains are fairly new to the cannabis market, many of them are just mixes of each other. The gene pool for CBD strains is currently not as diverse as that of high-THC strains.

High CBD strains do not produce that cloudy, mental haziness or paranoia associated with THC.

1. CBD Critical Cure

CBD Critical Cure is an excellent cannabis strain. Bred by Barney's Farm Seeds, this strain is a cross between Critical Kush and a ruderalis strain. Considered indica-dominant, inhaling this flower is like taking a breath of calm ease. Producing about a 2:1 ratio of CBD to THC, most CBD

Critical Cure buds feature around 11 percent CBD and 5 percent THC. The indica dominance of this strain makes it slightly sedative, which may be beneficial to those struggling to calm down on a difficult day. Consumers might experience a very slight psychoactive effect with this strain.

2. Harlequin

Harlequin is an excellent CBD strain. Featuring an almost 5:2 ratio of CBD to THC, this sativa does not generally produce a psychoactive high. Instead, Harlequin provides an ever so slightly energized and focused experience along with an easy mood uplift and anxiolytic (anti-anxiety) properties.

This unique flower has international heritage. A cross between Colombian, Thai, Swiss, and Nepalese landrace strains, the THC in Harlequin rarely exceeds 6 percent. The CBD in this flower can reach as high as 15 percent.

3. Sour Tsunami

Sour Tsunami is considered a one-to-one strain. That means that this flower tends to produce an even ratio of THC and CBD. The CBD in this bud may be slightly higher than the THC, often testing about 11 percent. THC averages about 10. A cross between Sour Diesel and New York Sour Diesel, this bud was one of the first high-CBD strains to become popular. Though some might experience some slight psychoactivity with this strain, Sour Tsunami provides a well-rounded and pleasant mood uplift.

4. Harle-tsu

Harle-tsu is a cross between the two equally famous high-CBD strains mentioned above: Harlequin and Sour

Tsunami. This flower is considered a high-CBD/low-THC strain. Harle-tsu often produces CBD levels that are almost 20 times higher than THC. Though, some phenotypes may produce more of a 1:1 ratio.

The result is a strain that produces no psychoactivity. Instead, this bud quietly eases anxiety and aids focus without really causing any noticeable change in cognitive function at all. Great for the day, this strain would be perfect for a vape break on a stressful day.

5. Stephen Hawking Kush

Stephen Hawking Kush is a cross between Harle-tsu and Sin City Kush. This strain is another one-to-one flower, often featuring about 5 percent CBD to 5 percent THC.

This flower is an excellent way to wind down without experiencing the paranoia or anxiety that is often associated with THC. Considered an indica, this bud has a relaxing quality to it, which may be beneficial to those who need to calm down during a panic.

6. Cannatonic

Cannatonic is a high CBD strain that features at least a 2:1 ratio of CBD to THC. A cross between two heavy indica strains, MK Ultra and G-13, this strain has a slight sedative quality. Like most CBD strains, Cannatonic promotes focus and may even help improve mental functioning in times of stress.

Typically, this strain expresses up to 17 percent CBD and around 6 percent THC. The higher the CBD, the less noticeable the foggy effects of THC will be.

7. ACDC

ACDC is a derivative of Cannatonic. The major difference is that this bud produces an almost 20 to 1 ratio of CBD to THC. This makes this strain more or less hemp. However, this flower can sometimes produce up to 6 percent THC. The CBD in this bud can reach a whopping 24 percent CBD.

Since CBD is a powerful anxiolytic, this strain may be particularly useful to those with more problematic anxiety disorders. ACDC does not produce a psychoactive high at all. Instead, it may provide feelings of alertness, focus, and serene mental clarity.

8. Canna-tsu

Similar to Harle-tsu, Canna-tsu is a true hybrid cross between Cannatonic and Sour Tsunami. Unlike Harle-tsu, Canna-tsu is generally considered to be a one-to-one strain. The THC in this bud might even be slightly higher than the CBD, often containing about 8 and 7 percent of each respective cannabinoid.

Since THC may be slightly higher, consumers may notice a slight psychoactivity from this bud. However, it's not quite right to say that Canna-tsu produces a "high." Rather, this earthy flower provides a calm yet uplifting and alert sensation that's perfect for just about any occasion.

9. CBD OG Kush

OG Kush is one of the most popular cannabis strains in history. The notoriously high THC strain now has a CBD match. CBD OG Kush is generally considered a one-to-one hybrid strain.

This bud is considered easy to grow and often features THC levels between 5 and 10 percent. The CBD this strain produces is about the same.

While Kushes are generally thought to cause some mental sedation, CBD OG Kush tends to have the opposite effect. In fact, some report that this strain can be quite alerting. Many CBD strains have similar effects, providing a mellow energy e□uivalent to sipping a calming cup of ginseng tea. CBD OG Kush is no different, making it excellent for the day.

10. CBD MediHaze

CBD MediHaze is considered a sativa-dominant hybrid. Like many CBD strains sold in medical and recreational cannabis dispensaries, CBD MediHaze features a fairly even ratio of THC to CBD. Both cannabinoids tend to run about 9 percent in this bud.

Inhaling a breath of CBD MediHaze is taking in a hit of sweet earth. A cross between Super Silver Haze and Neville's Haze, this strain produces a bright and crisp attention that is excellent for nerve-wracking events like public speaking and perhaps even for those who experience social anxiety.

Ways to enhance the anti-anxiety effects of CBD

CBD is a powerful anti-anxiety tool on its own. Yet, while many find CBD helpful, it works best when used in conjunction with therapy, nutritional, and appropriate medical support.

If you're hoping to get the most out of CBD for anxiety, here are a few ways to enhance the effects of the supplement:

1. Lavender

CBD is not the only plant compound with a calming effect.

While CBD may be unique in its ability to moderate memory and behavior, mixing it with other anxiolytic plant extracts may improve its anxiety-relieving abilities.

Research suggests that linalool, an aroma molecule most commonly found in lavender, has strong anxiolytic effects.

Some cannabis experts have suggested that combining CBD and linalool may have a beneficial and synergistic effect on anxiety.

Both CBD and lavender oil are available in tincture, oil, and capsule forms online.

2. Breathing techniques

In the midst of an anxiety attack, the body begins to produce excess amounts of the fight or flight hormone adrenaline.

This primes the body for an acute survival response.

When anxiety takes over, calming your physiology is an excellent emergency coping mechanism.

One of the fastest ways to calm your physiology is through deep breathing.

Taking a moment to consciously change your breathing patterns not only forces you to focus on something outside of your own thoughts but also helps transition the body to a calmer physical state.

3. Therapy

There is no doubt that many people feel that CBD produces genuine relief from anxiety.

However, CBD is only a helpful tool for overcoming anxiety, not a cure in and of itself.

Patients now have access to several different types of therapy that intend to create lasting relief by helping individuals change their fear patterns and behavior.

Cognitive behavioral therapy and exposure therapy are two popular forms of psychotherapy. Both types aim to help patients change patterns of thinking for an improved Quality of life in the long term.

CBD FOR INSOMNIA

Insomnia is a medical condition that nearly all of us go through at some point in our lives. This can be due to a wide range of reasons. However, it is treatable. And no, we're not suggesting you start taking sleeping pills. It is widely known that sleeping pills can be harmful to the human body, especially when it becomes a habit. A lack of sex drive as well as anxiety has been observed in people who frequently use sleeping pills. CBD, on the other hand, can be the answer to all your sleeping problems as it offers the best solution.

CBD for insomnia is a great choice. This is due to CBD's ability to regulate sleep cycles, helping to decrease activity in the brain and lead you to a restful, relaxed state of mind. For those with chronic insomnia, CBD proves to be a powerful cure especially if you would prefer not to take prescription drugs or sleep aids.

The benefits of CBD for sleep

CBD is becoming a more popular choice for insomnia as sufferers from sleeplessness struggle to find a cure. For many users of CBD, better sleep is a common benefit. This is due to CBD's many positive influences on the central nervous system, including greater relaxation and mood. As CBD tends to calm anxiety and generally help with the ability to sleep soundly, this powerful, natural agent should be considered one of the best ways to sleep fully and restfully during the night.

Anti-anxiety and PTSD

PTSD is a chronic psychiatric condition, that occurs due to an emotional trauma or fear triggered in the brain and can happen to any gender or age. Studies have concluded that CBD treats all form of anxiety including post-traumatic stress disorder and anxiety-provoked sleep disorder. As CBD has anti-inflammation properties, it keeps a check on radical stress and thus helps with better sleep.

Sleep Apnea

Sleep apnea is a serious sleep disorder when your breath repeatedly starts and stops. People who suffer from sleep apnea get repeatedly awakened by their own breathing because of the narrowed airway. Therefore, you feel tired even after a snoring sleep. This can cause high blood pressure, fatigue, diabetes, etc. Studies have revealed that CBD suppresses sleep apnea, as it is a muscle relaxant.

Chronic Pain

Waking up during the night and waking early due to chronic pain is a major sleep disruption. The problems with chronic pain get worse with insomnia and sleeping disorders. CBD might be the answer to this problem as it has been found useful to treat joint pain, arthritis, back pain, etc.

Depression

Feeling sad, lack of joy, reduced interest are all symptoms of the onset of depression. It is a mood disorder that causes lack of sleep. Causes of depression can be either genetic, environmental or psychological. A chemical imbalance in the brain is also a cause of depression. According to studies, CBD restores chemical balances in the brain by releasing serotonin; that is a natural mood stabilizer.

Thousands of people have given up their sleeping pills in favor of CBD. Taking CBD oil before bed and lifestyle changes can help you with a sound sleep.

How CBD affects sleep

There are many different cannabis extracts available. CBD is just one, with THC being the other. THC, as you know, cause the psychoactive effects of the cannabis plant. For this reason, it is not the best choice for relaxation and sleep.

However, CBD actually helps with decreasing brain activity, especially at night. In one study, done in 2006, it was found that CBD helped to stimulate restfulness, but it did not cause the paranoia or overactive imagination that sometimes results from THC. CBD works by activating certain compounds in the brain, leading to a sense of peace and positive mood.

Compounds in CBD that Boost Sleep

Within CBD, there is a specific compound that actually induces sleep. Some individuals who create CBD extracts use cannabis extracts that have been aged in order to get the most benefit from CBD sleep enhancing properties. Aged CBD compounds have been shown to be the most useful at promoting good sleep.

Benefits of CBD on the Brain

For individuals suffering from pain and physical ailments, CBD can be one of the best choices for helping you fall asleep. Through several recent studies, CBD has been shown to help alleviate symptoms of PTSD, MS, inflammation, muscular and joint dysfunction, and of course, insomnia. This is because CBD can help to relieve pain, which can prove to be a serious inhibitor of sleep. CBD can be taken as a pill or through inhaling, which is sometimes a more effective way of inducing a restful state. However, pills can act more quickly on the brain than inhalation methods, which is a consideration for those seeking a faster cure for insomnia from CBD.

CBD for Insomnia and Dreaming

Because CBD helps to create a more restful state of mind, dreaming can be better achieved through the use of this powerful agent. A study done on REM sleep while under the effect of CBD showed that users experienced more REM activity, while those who did not take cannabidiol were not able to achieve such effects.

Better Breathing with CBD

CBD has been shown to help those with asthma as well as sleep apnea. If you struggle with either of these problems, or simply can't seem to breathe soundly, regularly, and fully throughout the night, cannabidiol is a proven remedy. Some preclinical studies have shown that CBD helped over three-fourths of participants in a trial of CBD for breathing during sleep, largely due to the ability of cannabidiol to affect levels of serotonin in the brain. CBD is also able to reduce headaches and mood problems, which can also interfere with good breathing.

Improved Mood for Sleeping Soundly

One of the causes of insomnia is a racing mind or anxious thoughts while trying to fall asleep. Since CBD promotes positive mood through improved serotonin signaling as well as better dopamine levels, CBD for insomnia is undoubtedly one of the most effective ways to quickly get to sleep and stay that way. You will also find the benefits of CBD carrying through the rest of the day, in terms of better mood.

Since sound sleep can be one of the best ways to experience good moods throughout the day, CBD is considered an effective mood boosting remedy for all types of users. It is also holistic, natural, and safe, making it a good choice for those who wish to avoid non natural forms of insomnia relief.

HOW DO I TAKE CBD?

We have touched on the different ways to take CBD so far in this book. Now we're going to dive a little deeper and go into more depth. Most commonly, CBD is taken orally. This method is very easy to consume. It is discreet to use, and also it is very convenient to have a product that you can take on the go with you. In order to gain the most beneficial effects possible, you will want to look for a product that has various strains of CBD. This makes the product more potent and effective. There are many recommendations as far as dosage goes. One common method is to take 1-6mg per 10 pounds of body weight depending on your pain level. That's just a baseline. You can adjust up or down as your symptoms dictate. Although side effects are very rare, they can occur, such as dizziness, nausea or a headache. If these symptoms persist, you can stop the product or decrease the dosage. Many people experience an improvement in their symptoms after just one or two doses of CBD, but as with many products, you will find the best results occur after you have built the product up in your system a bit.

As time goes on, there is more and more research being done about CBD. Much of the findings that have already been procured, back the use of CBD as a therapeutic treatment, for many different conditions. Depending on what a person's current health status is, CBD may very well be effective in helping them lead a healthier and happier life.

It is beneficial to do your own research on CBD, rather than listening to other people's opinions. Many people are uneducated about CBD and assume it is the same thing as using marijuana or another drug. The effects of CBD are actually very beneficial and can help someone lead a very healthy life.

What steps should I take?

If you are thinking about starting up a regimen of CBD to embrace all of its potential health benefits, take some time to do your research. You'll want to think about what you want to accomplish in order to pick the right product.

- Do some initial research on hemp, CBD marijuana, what are CBDs, etc. Try to learn all that you can about these products. You'll be better educated on what your options are.
- It's always a good idea to talk to your doctor about CBD products. If you have been diagnosed with a medical condition of any sort, or if you are taking a prescription medication, you'll want to ensure there is no risk for interaction. Keep in mind that many medical professionals have strong opinions about cannabis in general and will not differentiate between CBD and THC or the hemp and marijuana cannabis plants.
- When shopping for CBD, your best option is the internet. This is where you can find the most

information, find the biggest variety of products and you have the ability to research the brands and distributors that you are considering. If you need to find out more about a potential product, contact the website or manufacturer of the product. If the lab test results on a particular brand of CBD isn't readily available on the website, don't be afraid to ask for it before you buy the product. There are many products out there that make claims that aren't true (snake oil).

- After receiving a product, read the dosing information thoroughly. Make sure that you understand how to take the product, how to store the product and if there are any side effects to watch out for.

- If you are thinking about increasing your dose, make sure you have waited for about three weeks before increasing the product. You'll want to wait about three weeks in between increases. This allows plenty of time for the product to build up in your system.

The consumption methods available for CBD

Concentrates

CBD concentrates are the most potent form of CBD in the market. It's not unusual for CBD concentrates to contain 10 times as much as the CBD found in other products. Concentrates are a great way to consume CBD if you are suffering from chronic illness, not just because of its potency but also because they are discreet, mess-free, and they only take a few seconds to set in. However, most CBD concentrates aren't flavored which can be discouraging for some users. CBD concentrates ideal for recreational or medical users re🞑uire a strong dose fast, especially when they are busy.

Tinctures

Tinctures are a popular way of consuming CBD. Just like concentrates, tinctures are a way to consume CBD in its purest form. There are some tinctures that have been created with flavors which make them more enjoyable to consume. Tinctures are taken sublingually, by placing a few drops just underneath your tongue. CBD tinctures in the market come in different dosages to suit different needs. The best way to get the most out of tinctures is by not swallowing the product as soon as you put it underneath your tongue; instead, place the drops sublingually and some on the sides of your cheeks and leave it for a few minutes.

Sprays

CBD sprays are consumed orally, by spraying the product directly into the mouth, underneath the tongue. They are usually weak in concentration although they offer the benefits of being portable, easy to use while traveling, and come in different flavors.

Edibles

CBD edibles are made from the same process that makes THC edibles, except they don't get you high. They come in many forms from savory to sweet treats and can be enjoyed by recreational as well as medical users. CBD edibles are preferred by patients suffering from inflammation, respiratory infections, chronic pain, insomnia, cancer, anxiety, and much more. The primary advantage of CBD edibles is that its effects last for a much longer time; on average, around 4-6 hours depending on the type of edible as well as the individual's biochemistry.

Capsules

Capsules are the most convenient way to take CBD daily as a supplement for health and prevention. They can be made at home or purchased online. CBD capsules typically contain around 10 to as much as 450mg of CBD, and if you feel that you need more CBD for a certain day you can just take 2 or more capsules. You can also use CBD capsules alongside other forms of CBD such as concentrates or tinctures for days that you need extra strength. All you need to do is swallow a capsule with water just like any other kind of nutritional supplement.

Topicals

Topicals are meant to be used for the skin, and are particularly beneficial for individuals suffering from eczema, psoriasis, chronic pain, arthritis, joint pain, acne, and other skin conditions. CBD topicals can also be used for its anti-aging properties. The cannabinoids are absorbed through CBD receptors found on the skin, allowing for localized relief.

Vapes

Vaping CBD oil is gaining popularity for its discretion and quick onset. It's also a great method for those who need total control over dosage. There are many ways to vape CBD oil like vape pens, vaporizers, and e-cigarettes. Heat and inhale – uick and easy. CBD oils made for vapes are also available in many delicious flavors, making the experience much more enjoyable.

Factors to take into account when calculating dosage

Administering CBD oil is similar to administering traditional medicines, so it's important to ensure that you take into account a few important factors when calculating your dose. Some things to consider are:

- Body Weight
- Metabolism
- Diet
- Tolerance to CBD
- Severity of illness
- Age
- Other Medications
- The type of products you are taking; oils, edibles or drinks

We'll provide some general guidelines regarding weight and suggested dosage, but keep in mind that your weight may change. This can cause the amount of CBD you need to change as well.

If you lose weight (because of a decrease in anxiety, depression, or psychosis), the CBD dosage might go down. If you gain weight (because of regaining your appetite or no longer being nauseated), the amount of CBD may increase. That's why it's important to record your progress so you can adjust things accordingly.

Other factors are not so easy to adjust. Metabolism doesn't really change unless you make a drastic alteration in your habits (going from a sedentary lifestyle to an active lifestyle, for example). In addition, you can't □uantify your metabolism, so it can be tricky to gauge the speed of your digestion. But, from experience, you probably know whether you have a fast metabolism or a slow metabolism.

How much CBD should you take?

This is always the question of the day. There are as many different dosing philosophies as there are brands of CBD. How much CBD you take depends, in large part, on the potency of the strain. Whether you're consuming cannabis for the first time or you've been doing it for years, we always recommend starting small and progressing slowly. This will give your body a chance to adapt to the CBD without any negative reactions. As mentioned earlier, a good rule of thumb is to take 1-6mg of CBD for every 10 pounds of body weight depending on your level of pain. From there you can adjust your dosage up or down according to your own results.

Below are a few more of the many ways to calculate dosage which will be explained indepth. Although I like to keep it as simple as possible and recommend the "1-6mg per 10 pounds" method, some prefer more specific instructions.

Another body weight method

The amount of CBD you need depends on how much you weigh. Below, we've produced a table of dosage suggestions based on your weight and the severity of your ailment (pain level). Use these as suggestions as a starting point and adjust your dosage up or down accordingly.

	86-150Ibs	151-240Ibs	>240Ibs
Pain			
None-Mild	12mg	18mg	22mg
Medium	15mg	22.5mg	30mg
Severe	18mg	27mg	45mg

CBD dosage calculator method

Each CBD oil product will have a different dosage amount and a different percentage of CBD per dose. Thankfully, all it takes is a bit of simple math and you can use these numbers (along with the starting dosage recommendations listed above) to find how much CBD oil to take to get the right amount of CBD. Here's how to do it.

First, read the label of your CBD oil of choice to find the serving suggestions. It will probably say something like:

Serving Size: X number of drops

Elsewhere on the label will be listed the amount of CBD (in milligrams) per serving. With that information, you can use our CBD dosage calculator method to find the dose that's just right for you.

To help you in this regard, we'll walk you through calculating your ideal dose using a hypothetical CBD oil.

Sample Calculation

Below is the serving size and amount of CBD per serving for our hypothetical CBD oil:

Serving Size: 10 drops

Amount Per Serving: 25 mg

From that information, we can write the following equivalency:

10 drops = 25 mg CBD

Now, let's say you are a 180-pound male with mild pain. Your starting dosage per the chart above would be 18 mg. Rather than take too much too soon, we can figure out how much CBD each drop contains by dividing 25 by 10.

25 divided by 10 = 2.5

So each drop of CBD oil contains 2.5 mg of CBD.

Now, we can take our starting dosage from the chart (18 mg) and divide it by 2.5 mg to find out how many drops we need.

18 divided by 2.5 = 7.2

It takes 7.2 drops to administer 18 mg of CBD. It's going to be nearly impossible to give yourself 0.2 of a drop, so round this number to 7. If the number after the decimal is five or higher, consider rounding up instead of down.

So, all you need to do is:

Find the serving size for your CBD oil (in this case, 10 drops).

Find the CBD in milligrams (mg) that serving size contains (in this case, 25 mg).

Determine the suggested starting dosage for your weight and condition.

Do a little simple math.

No complicated formulas. No fancy tools necessary.

CBD dosage simple calculation

CBD dosage can also be calculated using simple mathematics.

- Find the recommended serving size for your CBD oil.
- Find the CBD in milligrams that serving size contains.
- Determine the suggested starting dosage for your weight and condition.
- If you need to increase or decrease the serving size to reach your recommended dose, simply work out the milligrams per drop and use that increase to reach your desired milligram amount.

There are many ways to experience the healing of CBD. From vaping CBD oil to CBD gummies, the options are pretty much endless and dictated only by your preference.

Of course, dosage always depend on the strength of your product so if you switch between brands or forms of CBD, make sure you recalculate your dosage accordingly. For example, often CBD vape juice has quite a different strength to other products, so if you choose that method, be sure to do your calculations.

Recommended dosages for different conditions

- Multiple Sclerosis (MS) symptoms: Cannabis plant extracts containing 2.5-120 milligrams of a THC/CBD combination daily for 2-15 weeks.
- Sleep Disorders: 40mg-160mg of oral CBD.
- Schizophrenia: 40-1,280mg oral CBD daily.
- Glaucoma: A single sublingual (under the tongue) CBD dose of 20-40mg (>40 mg may increase eye pressure).

Synthetic pure CBD exists, and while that sounds like a great idea, at this stage it does not have the same broad-spectrum effects as natural CBD. Stick to organic hemp-based CBD for best results.

Can you overdose on CBD?

Using a calculator is a fantastic way to get the ideal dose tailored to your needs, but don't be worried about taking too much. You can't overdose on CBD. One of the reasons

CBD is so popular and relied on for many is its safe reputation.

Of course, it is possible to take too much CBD for your body to process and as a result your body can feel drowsy or lightheaded, especially if you are a new user. But there are no cases of anyone overdosing on CBD to the point of causing death.

The safest method is to stick to small dose as laid out by your CBD dosage calculator to err on the side of caution, and increase your dose from there if needed.

Remember good quality CBD oil has little to no THC in it so ensure you purchase a brand that explicitly says this. Overall, CBD oil is an extremely low-risk option, especially when compared to traditional pharmaceuticals

Similarly, your tolerance level can have a major effect on the amount of CBD you need. Tolerance is particularly stubborn and often re□uires weeks, months, or even years to change.

All of these factors should be considered, tweaked, and recorded as you work through the CBD dosage calculator.

CBD usage general guidelines

Overall CBD from hemp sources is super safe and effective. Follow these general guidelines to make sure that you have a stress-free experience with CBD.

- Take a smaller dose at first, which can be increased if needed.

- Ensure that CBD is right for your condition or symptoms.
- You can take CBD with or without food. Some studies have shown CBD absorption is increased when taken with foods containing fatty acids.
- Be aware CBD usage generally comes with few long-term effects, with cannabidiol wearing off after around 3-4 hours.

CBD dosage can be crucial to having an excellent CBD experience, so it's worth it to take some time to calculate your perfect dose. Remember, since everyone's body chemistry is different, you will have to find your own perfect dose.

To find just the right dosage for your situation, we highly recommend starting small. Remember, the least amount of medicine you can take to feel relief from your symptoms the better. Notice that this isn't the first time we've mentioned starting small and working your way up. It can save you some money.

Experiment with a certain dosage for three days to give your body time to react to the medication. Adjust the dosage up or down accordingly for the next three-day period. If you feel any discomfort from a dosage, decrease it immediately the next time you take the CBD oil. You can always increase gradually from there. This introductory period can last from 2-3 weeks, depending on body type and ailment.

Final thoughts on CBD dosage calculator

Whether you choose to use a traditional table dosage calculator or an online calculator, putting in the extra effort to measure your CBD is definitely worthwhile to reap the wonderful benefits of this healing natural alternative.

A way to take CBD in the morning

While there really is no perfect time to take CBD oil, morning is likely the most popular time people decide to incorporate their CBD supplement into their day, perhaps by mixing CBD Liquid into their coffee, their favorite smoothie, or as part of an acai bowl.

A new innovative way people are adding CBD to their breakfast is to infuse CBD liquid into their favorite all-natural honey, and then drizzle the sweet substance over a bowl of Greek yogurt oatmeal.

CBD Infused Honey over Greek Yogurt Oatmeal

Ingredients:

- ½ cup rolled oats
- ½ banana, sliced
- 1 cup water
- ¼ cup Greek yogurt
- ½ teaspoon ground cinnamon
- ¼ cup fresh berries
- Pinch of salt
- CBD-infused honey

Instructions:

- Stir together oats, banana, cinnamon, salt, and water in a microwave-safe bowl.
- Cook for 2 to 3 minutes, or until water is absorbed.
- Stir to evenly distribute ingredients.
- Allow to cool for about 3 minutes.
- Spoon Greek yogurt over the oatmeal and stir.
- Drizzle CBD-Infused honey over oatmeal.
- Top with fresh berries.

A way to take CBD in the afternoon

Although CBD, when taken in food, can start interacting with your endocannabinoid system within minutes to hours of use, many benefits of a stimulated system are not fully experienced right away. You may find that taking CBD in the middle of the day is beneficial for maintaining CBD levels.

At lunchtime, CBD can be blended into your favorite sauce or salad dressing. For a healthy, balancing meal, you can toss CBD-infused lemon-garlic salad dressing with a couscous and kale salad.

Couscous, Kale, and Cranberry Salad

Ingredients:

- 5 cups kale
- ½ cup couscous
- ½ cup water
- ¼ cup almonds, sliced
- ¼ cup dried cranberries

- ¼ cup CBD-Infused Lemon-Garlic Salad Dressing

Instructions:

- Wash kale. Chop and measure out five cups and add to a large bowl.
- Prepare couscous according to package instructions using water.
- Pour CBD-infused lemon-garlic salad dressing into bowl with couscous. Use your hands to massage the dressing into the kale.
- Stir in the almonds and dried cranberries just before serving.

A way to take CBD in the evening

Some CBD consumers have reported that CBD provides them with a "relaxed" or "calm" feeling, and therefore prefer to deliver CBD to their systems in the evening before bed.

With CBD Liquid, you can end your hectic day with the balancing properties of a homemade CBD-infused Mexican hot chocolate.

CBD-Infused Mexican Hot Chocolate

Ingredients:

- 6 (12-ounce) cans evaporated milk
- 4 teaspoons ground cinnamon
- 1 tablespoon vanilla extract
- 1 teaspoon ground nutmeg
- Pinch cayenne pepper

- 2 (12-ounce) bags semisweet chocolate chips
- ¾ teaspoon CBD Li☐uid per cup
- Cocoa powder, for serving

Instructions:

- In a saucepan over medium heat, whisk together milk, cinnamon, vanilla extract, and nutmeg.
- Add chocolate chips. Stir gently until chocolate is melted.
- Cover and turn heat to low for 5 minutes.
- Pour the hot chocolate into a cup. Stir in CBD Liquid. Top with a dusting of cocoa powder.

DRUG TESTS: WILL CBD SHOW UP?

A drug test, referred to as a drug screening, analyzes urine to detect the presence of illegal drugs or prescription medications. Different drug tests screen for different drugs, depending on the needs of those administering it. Drug tests can use urine, blood, hair, sweat, or saliva, with each providing its own advantages for screening, including time since use, minimum amount detected, and accuracy.

Drug tests have now become a common condition for employment, but they are also used as part of parole requirements, during substance abuse programs, and by sports organizations to test for prohibited substances.

These drug screens often test for more than just marijuana use. They can also detect the use of opioids, alcohol, cocaine, barbiturates, methamphetamine, and more. Depending on the drug, the amount and frequency of use, detection may be possible for a few hours to a few weeks.

Unfortunately, drug tests are more effective at detecting past drug use, rather than actual impairment, which has lead to criticism of the use of drug tests as a requirement for employment. This is especially true in states where recreational or medical marijuana use has been legalized. According to the Drug and Alcohol Testing Industry

Associations, employers drug test to provide safe work environments, identify and refer employees who have drug or alcohol problems, and even to comply with local, state, and federal regulations.

Does CBD show up on a drug test?

Concerned CBD lovers can breathe a sigh of relief if they are concerned about a CBD drug test. Legally, hemp CBD products must contain less than 0.3% THC. Many contain even less than that, hovering around the 0.1% range. This is less than one-third of the THC found in even the most minimal high-CBD/low-THC strain found in a cannabis dispensary. At this rate, you would have to consume very high daily doses of the compound to have the slightest risk of testing positive for THC metabolites. This would be most concerning for those taking over 1,000 to 2,000 milligrams of CBD hemp oil extract daily. Fortunately, those who are anxious about having trace amounts of THC in their system can always purchase a urine self-test for reassurance.

CBD isolates and CBD crystalline also won't garner a positive result on a drug test. CBD isolates and crystalline are purified forms of CBD.

These forms, although generally not as effective as whole-plant cannabis, contain up to 99.9 percent of the cannabinoid, meaning that it is highly unlikely that they will contain enough THC to test positive on a drug test with CBD products.

Although you will fail a drug test for cannabis if you consume THC. As we've stated several times in this book,

THC is the primary psychoactive in the cannabis plant. It's the compound that causes the classic cannabis "high" as well as bringing its own set of medicinal benefits.

The most common drug test is a urinalysis. Urinalysis checks urine for drug metabolites, not for a particular substance itself. A metabolite is a breakdown product made after the body processes a particular substance. Cannabis urinalysis checks for the presence of a THC metabolite called THC-COOH.

They do not test for CBD metabolites unless a test was specifically ordered to check for the presence of CBD metabolites in urine. Blood tests, saliva tests, and hair tests check for the same metabolite. While CBD can show up on a drug test if it is being specifically tested for, it is not standard practice to test for CBD nor its metabolites. In fact, there is not even a federal guideline for testing for the presence of CBD in government employees. Finding a private employer that mandates a test for CBD would be like stabbing your finger on a needle in a haystack, if any exists at all.

It is standard practice to test only for THC-COOH. This means that CBD would not show up on a standard drug test.

When to worry about CBD oil and drug tests

All that being said, the source and quantity of CBD may matter when taking a drug test. Why? Because some CBD products may contain small or trace amounts of THC. If you purchase a high CBD strain from an adult dispensary, the product likely contains at least 1% THC, and often more. When consumed repeatedly throughout the day and in high quantities, even this small amount of THC may be enough to show up on a drug test.

Using the U.S. federal standards for drug testing, most testing facilities will flag a positive urinalysis if urine contains over 50 nanograms of THC-COOH per milliliter of urine. However, different employers or testing centers may choose to test for different cutoff concentrations.

When it comes to CBD, on the other hand, it would be highly unusual for those using hemp CBD products or CBD isolates to test positive on a drug test.

CONCLUSION

CBD is becoming an interesting combination of popular holistic medicine, miracle cure, and a natural answer to synthetic drugs dominating modern medicine. With CBD, patients receive the promise of being in control of their ailments and are no longer feeling at the mercy of their treating physicians. This has turned out to be a particularly powerful message. Many patients use CBD oils freely for ailments both confirmed and self-diagnosed, and the rapid innovations with CBD products have been quite impressive. But while new CBD products keep entering the market virtually unchecked, effective regulatory control of these products has stayed far behind. As a result, unknown risks about long-term effects remain unaddressed, especially in vulnerable groups such as children, the elderly, and the chronically or terminally ill. It should be noted that this discussion goes well beyond CBD only, as new products containing additional cannabinoids like CBG, THCV, and acidic cannabinoids are following closely behind. We know even less about these compounds than about CBD, and very limited human safety data are available.

In the end, the decision to incorporate CBD into your life is a very personal decision. Your health is your most valuable asset, and decisions affecting your health should never be taken lightly.